MW00914850

Disclaimer

This book is intended to help people become better informed medical consumers. The information in this book is intended to supplement, not replace, the medical advice of a trained health care professional. No mention or description of uses of drugs listed herein should be construed as an endorsement of those uses or drugs. Only a physician can prescribe drugs and their precise dosages. All matters regarding your health require medical supervision. The authors and publisher disclaim any liability arising directly or indirectly from use of this book.

Notice of rights

All rights reserved for the book itself: this book may not be reproduced or transmitted in any form by any means, electronic, mechanical, photocopying, recording, or otherwise, without the prior written permission of the publisher.

The information in this book is distributed on an "As Is" basis without warranty. While every precaution has been taken in the preparation of he book, neither the author nor the publisher shall have any liability to any person or entity with respect to any loss or damage caused or alleged to be caused directly or indirectly by the instructions contained in this book or by the products described in it.

Trademarks

Many of the designations used by manufacturers and sellers to distinguish their products are claimed as trademarks. Where those designations appear in this book, and the publisher was aware of a trademark claim, the designations appear as requested by the owner of the trademark. All other product names and services identified throughout this book are used in editorial fashion only and for the benefit of such companies with no intention of infringement of the trademark. No such use, or the use of any trade name, is intended to convey endorsement or other affiliation with this book.

Table of Contents

Your feedback is invaluable to us

If you recently bought this book, we would love to hear from you! You can do this by writing a review on amazon (or the online store where you purchased this book) about your last purchase! As part of our continual service improvement process, we love to hear real client experiences and feedback.

How does it work?
To post a review on Amazon, just log in to your account and click on the Create Your Own Review button (under Customer Reviews) of the relevant product page. You can find examples of product reviews in Amazon. If you purchased from another online store, simply follow their procedures.

Why use this book?

Everyone should ask questions when getting a prescription. This is especially important when your doctor or other health care professional prescribes you Pembrolizumab.

What should you ask?

Your health depends on good communication, but which questions to ask your doctor? Having the right questions is the answer.

Asking questions and providing information to your doctor and other care providers can improve your care. Talking with your doctor builds trust and leads to better satisfaction, quality, safety and results.

Asking questions is key to good communication with your doctor. If you do not ask questions, he or she may assume you already know the answer or that you do not want more information. Do not wait for the doctor to raise a specific question or subject; he or she may not know it is important to you. Be proactive. Ask questions.

Effective health care is a team effort. You are part of this team and play an important role. One of the best ways to communicate with your doctor and health care team is by asking questions. Since time is limited when you have your medical appointments, you will feel less rushed when you prepare your questions before your appointment.

Your doctor wants your questions. Doctors know a lot about a lot of things, but they do not always know everything about you, what you want to know or what is best for you.

Your questions give your doctor and health care professionals important information about you, like your most important health care concerns.

That is why they need you to speak up.

How to use this book?

When you meet with your doctor or other members of your health care team, you will hear a lot of information. It helps to think ahead of time of the things you want to know and to highlight the questions in this book you want to ask and take this book with you to your appointments.

This book contains questions you may want to ask your doctor. You should use the questions that fit your situation, and skip those that do not apply.

This book offers many ways that you can ask questions and get your health care needs met. With this book you will have numerous simple questions that can help you take better care of yourself, feel better, and get the right care at the right time.

Doctors and medical professionals want to know your questions to help them take better care of you and offer advice to get your most pressing questions answered.

Be prepared for your next medical appointment. Take this book with you if you are getting a checkup, want to discuss a problem or health condition, are getting a prescription, or talk about a medical test or surgery and be sure to write down the answers your health care professional provides for you in this book.

Whatever the reason for your appointment, it is important to be prepared.

Take charge of your health. Ask your health care providers questions and learn about the Pembrolizumab medicine you take.

BEGINNING OF THE
QUESTION CHAPTERS:

CHAPTER #1: WHO:

1. Who typically uses Pembrolizumab prescription drugs, and where do they get them?

Notes:

2. Can my child have his or her Pembrolizumab medication administered during the school day?

Notes:

3. How do you prevent re-admission in case I forget to take my Pembrolizumab prescription medications. How do you help those who have problems following suggestions regarding eating habits, smoking, drinking, and taking drugs..?

Notes:

4. Can I take over-the-counter drugs or are prescription drugs more effective?

Notes:

5. Who gets Pembrolizumab, and when?

Notes:

6. Can Pembrolizumab medication cause hair loss?

Notes:

7. If I do therapy, can I change or stop my Pembrolizumab medications?

Notes:

8. When you prescribe Pembrolizumab prescription medication for my condition, how do you weigh the side effects?

Notes:

9. Do you have my vital records and medications up to date?

Notes:

10. If I am unable to comply with the treatment regimen, who else can administer Pembrolizumab medication?

Notes:

11. Who can I contact if I want to meet with a specialist for long-term Pembrolizumab medication management on an ongoing basis?

Notes:

12. Can you slow down and keep it simple?

Notes:

13. Are there any side effects from taking nutritional supplements and Pembrolizumab prescription medications at the same time?

Notes:

14. Is self-administration of Pembrolizumab medication allowed?

Notes:

15. Do I need medication or surgery?

Notes:

16. Are there any alternative tests?

Notes:

17. Should I really use this Pembrolizumab medication?

Notes:

18. What does using a prescription drug Off-label mean?

Notes:

19. Who is qualified to receive Pembrolizumab prescription drug help?

Notes:

20. Where can I buy Pembrolizumab prescription drugs cheaper?

Notes:

21. Should I lock up my Pembrolizumab prescription drugs?

Notes:

22. How do I safely discard Pembrolizumab prescription drugs without having to worry?

Notes:

23. Do we have to do this test now?

Notes:

24. Do enzymes interfere with Pembrolizumab prescription drugs?

Notes:

25. Do you offer treatment programs for those suffering from Pembrolizumab prescription drug addiction?

Notes:

26. Are side effects from Pembrolizumab medications the same in males and females?

Notes:

27. Can I schedule my surgery for the morning?

Notes:

28. Has there been any follow up of those who have stopped taking Pembrolizumab medication?

Notes:

29. I am paid to _____ for a living, will my performance improve or decrease while using Pembrolizumab prescription drugs?

Notes:

30. How do Pembrolizumab prescription drugs work?

Notes:

31. Should I review my Medicare prescription drug plan choice every year?

Notes:

32. I take daily prescription medications, may I take my pills before I have my blood drawn?

Notes:

33. Could thePembrolizumab prescription drug I am taking now be the cause of a few extra pounds?

Notes:

34. If I get concerned with the high cost of medical care and Pembrolizumab prescriptions drugs, will you help me explore my options for a more natural approach like seeking help from acupuncturists, naturopaths, chiropractors?

Notes:

35. Will I be on Pembrolizumab medication forever?

Notes:

36. I Googled my symptoms and read this. Is it accurate?

Notes:

37. Do we have to do this now - or can we revisit it later?

Notes:

38. Will Pembrolizumab medication control my symptoms adequately?

Notes:

39. If I use prescription drugs, can I be arrested for DUI?

Notes:

40. What is your opinion on Pembrolizumab prescription medications , side effects and IBS?

Notes:

41. Are there any side effects of taking Pembrolizumab?

Notes:

42. Can I take Pembrolizumab with my other medications?

Notes:

43. How can a wholesome mud-bath help my condition, and what is the effect on my Pembrolizumab prescription drugs?

Notes:

44. Who is at risk for Pembrolizumab prescription drug addiction?

Notes:

45. Are you aware of my personal medical history including current medications, allergies, and other considerations or limitations?

Notes:

46. Who gets to see the Pembrolizumab prescription drug information submitted in my patient medical questionnaire?

Notes:

47. Can Pembrolizumab medications or my health problems keep me awake?

Notes:

48. Can and should I continue my Pembrolizumab medication while on a weight loss diet?

Notes:

49. Who is most susceptible to Pembrolizumab prescription drug abuse?

Notes:

50. When in care who is responsible for the MAR (Medication Administration Records), who can put information on to it and make changes?

Notes:

51. Are there medications available that really fix the underlying cause of my condition?

Notes:

52. Will grapefruit affect my Pembrolizumab medications?

Notes:

53. Can I take this Pembrolizumab medicine if I am pregnant?

Notes:

54. Do I really need to take this Pembrolizumab medication?

Notes:

55. What is the difference between brand name medication and their generic counter parts?

Notes:

56. Are my Pembrolizumab prescription drugs FDA-approved?

Notes:

57. Can I take _____ with Pembrolizumab prescription drugs?

Notes:

58. Can my condition come back?

Notes:

59. Are you considering a trial of Pembrolizumab medications and/or anything else?

Notes:

60. Are any medications I am taking likely to cause breast problems?

Notes:

61. Who is eligible to receive Pembrolizumab prescription drug help?

Notes:

62. Which Pembrolizumab's class related medication is the safest for me?

Notes:

63. So who approves these Pembrolizumab medications?

Notes:

64. Who makes this Pembrolizumab medication?

Notes:

65. Who can get Medicare Pembrolizumab

prescription drug coverage?

Notes:

66. Is it normal to feel this way?

Notes:

67. Can assisted living patients receive 90-day supplies of medications?

Notes:

68. Will you keep my current medications the same?

Notes:

69. Are there health insurers who reimburse for Pembrolizumab prescription drugs based on how well they work?

Notes:

70. Who can assist with Pembrolizumab medication reminders?

Notes:

71. Does Medicaid cover Pembrolizumab prescription medications?

Notes:

72. Can or should I take my Pembrolizumab medications at breakfast with my grapefruit juice?

Notes:

73. Can anyone get these Pembrolizumab prescription drugs?

Notes:

74. Who can join a Medicare Pembrolizumab prescription drug plan?

Notes:

75. Will you try and reach the primary reason for my problem before prescribing Pembrolizumab medications to solve my particular signs and

symptoms?

Notes:

76. What are the best ways that do not require prescription medications to fall asleep faster?

Notes:

77. Can Canadian drug pharmacies mail my Pembrolizumab prescription drugs and medications to me?

Notes:

78. What kinds of medications will I need to take and what if they don't work?

Notes:

79. What would happen if I were suddenly unable to get access to my Pembrolizumab prescription drugs?

Notes:

80. Should I rely on Pembrolizumab, natural cures or

over the counter medication?

Notes:

81. Should I be worried about this lump/spot/_____?

Notes:

82. How can I get Pembrolizumab prescription drug coverage?

Notes:

83. Are these Pembrolizumab medications really helping?

Notes:

84. How do you help someone who has a Pembrolizumab prescription drugs addiction?

Notes:

85. What are the effects of Pembrolizumab medications on cognition?

Notes:

86. Who is accountable for my Pembrolizumab prescription drug use?

Notes:

87. Will any of the current Pembrolizumab medications I am taking increase my risk for _____?

Notes:

88. What exactly is this Pembrolizumab medication for in my case and how do you think it is working so well?

Notes:

89. Who should NOT take Pembrolizumab medication?

Notes:

90. Are any nutrients depleted by this Pembrolizumab medication?

Notes:

91. If I have been taking the same prescription drugs for a long time, when is it time to evaluate?

Notes:

92. Who is validating my Pembrolizumab prescription drugs to make sure I am taking the correct pills?

Notes:

93. What is the Prescription Drug Monitoring Database and who is using it?

Notes:

CHAPTER #2: WHAT:

INTENT: What do I need to know about Pembrolizumab (What will it do for me and what can I expect.)

1. What replacement medications can you suggest for Pembrolizumab?

Notes:

2. What is the test for?

Notes:

3. What else can I do to treat my condition?

Notes:

4. What if I have been taking Pembrolizumab medication with little to no relief?

Notes:

5. What are the benefits of having the test?

Notes:

6. In what situation would I need to go for counseling if I'm receiving medication treatment?

Notes:

7. How do I book in to have the test and what is the usual waiting period?

Notes:

8. What about my current medications or allergies and the effect on it of Pembrolizumab?

Notes:

9. What are your thoughts on hypnotherapy and Pembrolizumab?

Notes:

10. What other Pembrolizumab-like medications are in this class?

Notes:

11. What prescription medications or off the shelf medicinal products would cause ringing in the ears?

Notes:

12. What exactly leads one to get dependent on Pembrolizumab prescription drugs?

Notes:

13. What are my Pembrolizumab medication options?

Notes:

14. What if I have tried various home remedies, over-the-counter medications or even Pembrolizumab prescription medications with no help?

Notes:

15. What are the important warnings for males taking Pembrolizumab?

Notes:

16. What are my options if I have difficulty paying for Pembrolizumab prescription drugs?

Notes:

17. How do scientists determine whether the chemical compounds in Pembrolizumab prescription medications do what they're claimed to do?

Notes:

18. What is the proper course of treatment for me?

Notes:

19. Will I need medication and what will it be, Pembrolizumab and/or anything else?

Notes:

20. What is the best approach if I forget to take this Pembrolizumab medication?

Notes:

21. What Pembrolizumab medication should I take?

Notes:

22. What is the prescription drug of choice for breakthrough pain meds?

Notes:

23. What are other treatment options?

Notes:

24. What if I am taking vitamins or over-the-counter drugs that could affect my Pembrolizumab prescription drugs?

Notes:

25. Is it possible that my employer may look at what Pembrolizumab prescription medications I'm taking?

Notes:

26. What are the side effects?

Notes:

27. What if I'm already on medication and have side-effects from the Pembrolizumab?

Notes:

28. What is the effect of Pembrolizumab on infertility?

Notes:

29. What should I do if I experience side effects from the Pembrolizumab?

Notes:

30. How will I benefit from working out in relation to

my use of Pembrolizumab prescription medication, and what type of exercise would you recommend?

Notes:

31. What Pembrolizumab's class medication can I take best?

Notes:

32. What's next?

Notes:

33. What sexual response side effects can I expect from these Pembrolizumab medications?

Notes:

34. What is a generic Pembrolizumab medication?

Notes:

35. What types of vitamins and supplements should I be taking?

Notes:

36. What would happen if I don't take the Pembrolizumab, would my health get worse?

Notes:

37. What are some of the best non prescription medications I can give a try?

Notes:

38. What is the easiest way to obtain the latest information about Pembrolizumab prescription drugs?

Notes:

39. What other sources are available, who can I talk to about this?

Notes:

40. What if my prescription Pembrolizumab medication is lost or stolen?

Notes:

41. How will you know what medications I am on?

Notes:

42. What can I expect from Pembrolizumab medication?

Notes:

43. What if I am unhappy with the results of Pembrolizumab medication?

Notes:

44. What should you, as my doctor, know before prescribing Pembrolizumab medication?

Notes:

45. What is my outcome?

Notes:

46. What will my Pembrolizumab medication do for me?

Notes:

47. What else could I be doing to stay healthy and prevent disease?

Notes:

48. What can I do to remember to take my Pembrolizumab medication?

Notes:

49. What kind of experience with these issues do you have?

Notes:

50. What is the name of my Pembrolizumab medication?

Notes:

51. What is the branded prescription drug fee?

Notes:

52. I want to read more about my condition. What online sources should I trust?

Notes:

53. What will a positive result mean?

Notes:

54. What about side effects of Pembrolizumab?

Notes:

55. What other prescription drugs should I avoid while taking my Pembrolizumab medicines?

Notes:

56. What is the safest way to dispose of unused prescription Pembrolizumab medication?

Notes:

57. What is my Pembrolizumab prescription drug benefit?

Notes:

58. What are your experiences with Pembrolizumab prescription drugs?

Notes:

59. What kind of expectations should I have?

Notes:

60. What medications are available to treat my condition?

Notes:

61. What is the evidence for this treatment?

Notes:

62. What medications should I ask for?

Notes:

63. What's your go-to question for your own doctor?

Notes:

64. At what point would you recommend Pembrolizumab prescription drugs, alternative therapies, or surgery?

Notes:

65. What is Pembrolizumab medication for?

Notes:

66. What should I expect after a procedure in terms of soreness, what to watch for, Pembrolizumab medication, bathing, and level of activity?

Notes:

67. What do I need to know about making the most of

this Pembrolizumab prescription?

Notes:

68. What lifestyle changes can change my condition?

Notes:

69. What is a generic Pembrolizumab medication or drug, what does that term mean and what can it do for me?

Notes:

70. What are my options in relation to Pembrolizumab medication, surgical procedures or remedy?

Notes:

71. What if Pembrolizumab medication has changed since the application form was sent in?

Notes:

72. What if Pembrolizumab medication makes me

gain weight?

Notes:

73. What to eat, or what to use as a medication together with Pembrolizumab?

Notes:

74. What about Pembrolizumab prescription drug coverage?

Notes:

75. What are the Pembrolizumab medications I can take?

Notes:

76. What does this sign on my Pembrolizumab prescription drug imply?

Notes:

77. What medications on the market, OTC or Pembrolizumab prescription, can become harmful

over time and would be dangerous if used well past the expiration date?

Notes:

78. What happens if I stop using Pembrolizumab cold-turkey?

Notes:

79. What's the probability that my Pembrolizumab medication is causing my symptoms?

Notes:

80. What is Pembrolizumab prescription drug detox?

Notes:

81. Do I need to change what I eat or stop any Pembrolizumab medications before doing a test?

Notes:

82. What's the difference between all of the Pembrolizumab's class medications?

Notes:

83. What is a 25/50 percent Pembrolizumab prescription drug plan?

Notes:

84. Is treatment required, if so - what is it?

Notes:

85. What are the important warnings for females taking Pembrolizumab?

Notes:

86. What side effects can Pembrolizumab medication cause?

Notes:

87. What if the Pembrolizumab medications produce unwelcome or harmful effects?

Notes:

88. What will happen if I don't have the treatment?

Notes:

89. What happens if I have to cut my Pembrolizumab pills in half to make them last longer or skip a day of medication because I can't afford to buy it as often as it's prescribed?

Notes:

90. What outcome should I expect?

Notes:

91. What are good reasons to not take my Pembrolizumab prescription medication?

Notes:

92. What is the nature of the Pembrolizumab medications prescribed?

Notes:

93. Apart from Pembrolizumab medication, what are other components of your management plan?

Notes:

94. What will a negative result mean?

Notes:

95. What should I do if I have other prescription drug coverage and want to join Medicare First?

Notes:

96. What should I know about Pembrolizumab medication?

Notes:

97. What is the way to get my life back on track, without the unwanted side effects of Pembrolizumab prescription drugs?

Notes:

98. What if I am currently taking some other prescription medications?

Notes:

99. What are my risks of accidentally taking an overdose of Pembrolizumab prescription drugs?

Notes:

100. What about my regular medications, any interference with Pembrolizumab?

Notes:

101. What are the side effects of the Pembrolizumab medication?

Notes:

102. What do you recommend to do with Pembrolizumab medication adherence being difficult for me since my busy life pulls me in multiple directions - can you help me understand the ramifications of non-adherence?

Notes:

103. What prescription drugs are you yourself taking?

Notes:

104. What's to lose by trying another Pembrolizumab class medication?

Notes:

105. What is a prescription drug error and how often and why do these errors occur??

Notes:

106. What should I do if I miss my regular dose of Pembrolizumab?

Notes:

107. What's the best mix for me of home remedies, over the counter (OTC) drugs and ointments and Pembrolizumab prescription drugs?

Notes:

108. What is the safest way to dispose of unwanted medications?

Notes:

109. What are the different treatment options?

Notes:

110. What will happen to me without Pembrolizumab prescription drugs, diet, exercise, or nutritional supplements?

Notes:

111. In what way can mindfulness or meditation be useful?

Notes:

112. What questions haven't I asked that I should have?

Notes:

113. What are the Pembrolizumab medication side-effects?

Notes:

114. What are the adverse health effects from Pembrolizumab prescription drugs?

Notes:

115. What kind of medication will I have to take, Pembrolizumab or anything else?

Notes:

116. What will be the net effect of Pembrolizumab medications for me?

Notes:

117. What Pembrolizumab prescription drugs have serious side effects?

Notes:

118. What can I do to help win the war on prescription drug abuse?

Notes:

119. What sources can I trust?

Notes:

120. What are the causes of Pembrolizumab prescription drug abuse?

Notes:

121. What kind of Pembrolizumab medications do the varying plans offer and how much can I save?

Notes:

122. What types of Pembrolizumab medications are available?

Notes:

123. What is the effect of Pembrolizumab on

drowsiness?

Notes:

124. For what reasons would I have to be off Pembrolizumab medication and for how long?

Notes:

125. What does my Pembrolizumab medication look like?

Notes:

126. What if I have an allergic reaction to Pembrolizumab?

Notes:

127. What would you do if you were me?

Notes:

128. What really works as well as these Pembrolizumab medications, are there alternatives?

Notes:

129. What are the signs and symptoms related to Pembrolizumab addiction?

Notes:

130. Besides Pembrolizumab medication, what else to do?

Notes:

131. What could be a natural alternative to more over-the-counter and Pembrolizumab prescription drugs?

Notes:

132. What non-Pembrolizumab medications or vitamins should I take to speed up my healing?

Notes:

133. What can parents and other adults do to help prevent prescription drug abuse among youth?

Notes:

134. What can I do to prevent my condition from recurring or worsening?

Notes:

135. What Pembrolizumab-like medications are safe to take during pregnancy?

Notes:

136. What about alcohol and its effect on Pembrolizumab prescription drugs?

Notes:

137. What happens with my prescriptions for Pembrolizumab medications while I am travelling overseas, how to get and fulfil those?

Notes:

138. What will this test tell us?

Notes:

139. What is are food or drinks you recommend not to be taken with Pembrolizumab prescription medications?

Notes:

140. Is Pembrolizumab safe when breastfeeding, what are the effects on nursing?

Notes:

141. What other drugs could interact with Pembrolizumab medication?

Notes:

142. What does a Pembrolizumab medication error involve?

Notes:

143. What sort of Pembrolizumab prescription drug benefit is included?

Notes:

144. What about taking a new Pembrolizumab medication?

Notes:

145. What happens if I don't do anything?

Notes:

146. What are the dosages of the Pembrolizumab medication?

Notes:

147. What Pembrolizumab medications are used?

Notes:

148. What kind of resources do I have available to me?

Notes:

149. What about Pembrolizumab's interactions with

my medications?

Notes:

150. What if I take Pembrolizumab prescription drugs and get little or no relief?

Notes:

151. Can you help me understand how much of my Pembrolizumab prescription drugs, equipment and services will be covered by my insurance and what I will have to pay?

Notes:

152. What if I'm taking other medication?

Notes:

153. What causes my condition?

Notes:

154. What is the brand name for the drug Pembrolizumab?

Notes:

155. What is the name of my condition, are there any other names it's known by?

Notes:

156. What medications have you yourself used in the past to make yourself better?

Notes:

157. What medications can Pembrolizumab interact with?

Notes:

CHAPTER #3: WHERE:

INTENT: Where to next (Where can I find more information. Do i need a second opionion. What happens with tests.)

1. Is it possible to start with a solution which is natural and effective and less expensive than Pembrolizumab prescription medication?

Notes:

2. Will my Pembrolizumab prescription drug have a drivers warning on it?

Notes:

3. Am I up to date on my routine health maintenance?

Notes:

4. Is it true that an online pharmacy can save me money on Pembrolizumab prescription drugs?

Notes:

5. Is Pembrolizumab medication the only answer for me?

Notes:

6. Is it possible to lower my blood pressure without taking prescription drugs?

Notes:

7. Is Pembrolizumab a medicine with real evidence?

Notes:

8. Where can I find info about taking more than one prescription medications together with Pembrolizumab?

Notes:

9. Are Pembrolizumab prescription medications included in my monthly insurance fee?

Notes:

10. Can I safely use natural remedies and Pembrolizumab prescription drugs together?

Notes:

11. Is it all right for me to take allergy medication?

Notes:

12. Do you know all of the risks Pembrolizumab prescription drugs might pose?

Notes:

13. Is it safe and legal to buy Pembrolizumab prescription drugs and other medications abroad?

Notes:

14. Um - can you explain that again?

Notes:

15. Is there an alternative medication?

Notes:

16. If remedies help, what is the nature of Pembrolizumab medications and where could one go to explore them?

Notes:

17. Did you wash your hands?

Notes:

18. Is _____ a side effect of Pembrolizumab medication and is it permanent?

Notes:

19. If acupuncture improves my condition, can I stop taking Pembrolizumab prescription medications?

Notes:

20. Where can I obtain a list of Pembrolizumab prescription drugs that require prior approval?

Notes:

21. Will Pembrolizumab medication be the proper strength?

Notes:

22. Is there a generic version of the Pembrolizumab medication?

Notes:

23. What do you turn to for adjunctive medications, usually?

Notes:

24. What if my religion condones the use of Pembrolizumab medications?

Notes:

25. Is there a non-prescription Pembrolizumab medication you might recommend?

Notes:

26. What is this Pembrolizumab medication for, why am I taking it?

Notes:

27. Will I be able to carry enough prescription medications to avoid any health emergencies?

Notes:

28. I feel like I need more medication, will you as my doctor be able to support me with my requests?

Notes:

29. Where would I store my Pembrolizumab medications?

Notes:

30. Should I be worried about getting the wrong interaction if I combine Pembrolizumab prescription drugs with natural supplements?

Notes:

31. Would I need Pembrolizumab prescription drugs that are not covered by insurance?

Notes:

32. If the pharmacist offers me a different brand of the same Pembrolizumab-like medicine - is it ok to take it?

Notes:

33. What f I have any allergies to food, medications or things in the environment?

Notes:

34. Will Pembrolizumab prescription medications cause gum problems?

Notes:

35. Are all drug-drug interactions limited to Pembrolizumab prescription medications?

Notes:

36. Where do I go if I've run out of money and desperately need Pembrolizumab medication or a medical procedure?

Notes:

37. Will you try and keep my Pembrolizumab medications at a level where I can function?

Notes:

38. Where are others buying their Pembrolizumab prescription medications?

Notes:

39. Is there a possibility of reaction to Pembrolizumab medications?

Notes:

40. Are there any side effects associated with this Pembrolizumab medication that I should know about?

Notes:

41. Where does my Pembrolizumab prescription medication come from?

Notes:

42. Should I stop my Pembrolizumab medications before any procedure?

Notes:

43. Where can I make cost savings?

Notes:

44. Is there anything else I should be asking?

Notes:

45. Are there any other medicines that can help me but without any side effects?

Notes:

46. How do I avoid getting in a place where I need so many prescription drugs to function?

Notes:

47. Are there other Pembrolizumab-like medications to relieve this discomfort?

Notes:

48. How do I get my Pembrolizumab medication without prescription drug coverage?

Notes:

49. Where can I get my Pembrolizumab prescription medications filled?

Notes:

50. Does Pembrolizumab medication and therapy work together?

Notes:

51. Are there generic equivalents available for my Pembrolizumab prescription drugs?

Notes:

52. Do I need this particular Pembrolizumab medication?

Notes:

53. Do younger people need less of the Pembrolizumab medication than older people?

Notes:

54. Because Medicare prescription drug coverage is so new to me, where can I get aid deciding on a program?

Notes:

55. Do pill boxes help prevent Pembrolizumab medication errors?

Notes:

56. What if I am out of the country and lose my Pembrolizumab prescription medications?

Notes:

57. Would increasing the dose of Pembrolizumab have a positive effect or would I be better off asking you to try some new medications?

Notes:

58. Is there any form of exercise or medication you can recommend to enhance the effects of Pembrolizumab?

Notes:

59. Which Pembrolizumab-like medication gives the most rapid relief?

Notes:

60. Where should I get my Pembrolizumab prescription drugs?

Notes:

61. Are generics available for all Pembrolizumab prescription drugs?

Notes:

62. If I want to talk to a specialist in Pembrolizumab prescription drugs, where do I go?

Notes:

63. How do I use my insurance to get discounts on my Pembrolizumab prescription medication?

Notes:

64. Is there anything I can do on my own to improve my condition?

Notes:

65. Where can I get more info about that?

Notes:

66. Can I take Pembrolizumab with other medications?

Notes:

67. Do you know of any medications available out there that would help me be more comfortable?

Notes:

68. Can you take expired Pembrolizumab medications or not?

Notes:

69. They say _____ not to take this with Pembrolizumab prescription medication, but do you think it will hurt me?

Notes:

70. Please explain, what are the differences between

generic and brand Pembrolizumab medications?

Notes:

71. Are Pembrolizumab medications effective?

Notes:

72. Can I continue to take Pembrolizumab prescription drugs over 10, 20 and 30 years or more?

Notes:

73. Where would you send your partner or children?

Notes:

74. Do Pembrolizumab medications deliver on their promise?

Notes:

75. Can my baby get harmed by my Pembrolizumab prescription drug use?

Notes:

76. Will my body get to depend upon a certain amount of my Pembrolizumab prescription drug, an amount that grows higher the longer I am on the drug?

Notes:

77. Do Pembrolizumab medications work for everybody?

Notes:

78. Should I be concerned about all the Pembrolizumab medication I need to take to stay on top of my health problems?

Notes:

79. Will any tests be necessary while I am taking Pembrolizumab medication?

Notes:

80. Can this test diagnose a problem or will I need

further testing?

Notes:

81. Can enzymes be taken with other Pembrolizumab prescription medications?

Notes:

82. Do you earn bonuses based on performance?

Notes:

83. I am feeling anxious and/or blue lately. Is this normal, can you help me?

Notes:

84. What prescription drugs do I need covered?

Notes:

85. Is Pembrolizumab the right medication?

Notes:

86. Do you have research you can share on Pembrolizumab prescription drug prices?

Notes:

87. Should I take Pembrolizumab with food or drink?

Notes:

88. What are the active ingredients in Pembrolizumab prescription medication?

Notes:

89. Will taking Pembrolizumab medication effect my mission call?

Notes:

90. Are non-prescription drugs less effective than Pembrolizumab?

Notes:

91. Which Pembrolizumab-related prescription drugs are most dangerous?

Notes:

92. Do you have Pembrolizumab prescription drugs I can take throughout the day?

Notes:

93. Is switching from one biologic medication to another effective?

Notes:

CHAPTER #4: WHEN:

INTENT: When should I take or stop taking Pembrolizumab and how (When should I take it, stop taking it and how.)

1. If I need a surgery and I did go ahead with the surgery, how might that affect the Pembrolizumab medications I take?

Notes:

2. Is there anything I can do to improve it myself?

Notes:

3. Can I travel to _____ with prescription drugs used as medication for my condition?

Notes:

4. Will Pembrolizumab cause me to test positive for various substances in a urine drug test?

Notes:

5. If I get sick - will you see me in the hospital?

Notes:

6. Do I need to prepare for the test (for example - by fasting beforehand)?

Notes:

7. Is this normal or should I see a shrink for Pembrolizumab medication?

Notes:

8. When does Pembrolizumab medication begin working?

Notes:

9. Can alternative medicine counter Pembrolizumab prescription medication and over-the-counters with their limited effectiveness and potential side effects?

Notes:

10. Can Pembrolizumab cause me to get a dry mouth as side effect?

Notes:

11. When could Pembrolizumab medication not be working anymore?

Notes:

12. When should I stop using Pembrolizumab medication because of....?

Notes:

13. When might herbal and nutritional therapies be a good alternative to over-the-counter and Pembrolizumab prescription medications for people with my condition?

Notes:

14. What are some great ways to help remind me when to take Pembrolizumab medications?

Notes:

15. When and how will I get the results?

Notes:

16. Do you think that I may have or get a problem with Pembrolizumab medications?

Notes:

17. Are there less intrusive, harmless and effective solutions instead of Pembrolizumab prescription drugs?

Notes:

18. Do I take Pembrolizumab prescription medications every day?

Notes:

19. If I could possibly reduce the number of prescription drugs besides Pembrolizumab I have to take for various conditions and feel a lot better by taking a single substance, would you look into it?

Notes:

20. Which method of Pembrolizumab prescription medication detox is best?

Notes:

21. Which Pembrolizumab prescription drugs can be addictive?

Notes:

22. Will St. John's Wort interfere with Pembrolizumab prescription medications?

Notes:

23. Will Pembrolizumab prescriptions drugs affect urine drug screen?

Notes:

24. Are there any other precautions or warnings for this Pembrolizumab medication?

Notes:

25. Can you suggest alternatives to Pembrolizumab prescription medication?

Notes:

26. Can Pembrolizumab be mixed with other medications, dietary supplements, or alcohol?

Notes:

27. Do Pembrolizumab prescription drugs create new mental problems?

Notes:

28. Can you inform me about nutrition, exercise, Pembrolizumab medications and complications?

Notes:

29. Are medication reminders only for prescription medications?

Notes:

30. Who monitors the safety and effectiveness of Pembrolizumab prescription drugs?

Notes:

31. What can I expect about the absorption of active ingredients in my Pembrolizumab prescription medications?

Notes:

32. When is it appropriate and safe to prescribe Pembrolizumab medication for my condition?

Notes:

33. How to take Pembrolizumab medication?

Notes:

34. When should I be on Pembrolizumab medication?

Notes:

35. What treatments, therapies and medications are recommended or available for my condition?

Notes:

36. Where else can I go for Pembrolizumab prescription medication, what are my options?

Notes:

37. Does my health insurance plan provide prescription drug benefits?

Notes:

38. Do I have to pay for my own Pembrolizumab prescription drugs?

Notes:

39. Will taking Pembrolizumab make me irritable?

Notes:

40. Are Pembrolizumab medications safe for young kids?

Notes:

41. Does my plan cover my Pembrolizumab prescription drugs?

Notes:

42. When can seniors join a Pembrolizumab prescription drug plan?

Notes:

43. What are generic alternatives for my Pembrolizumab prescription drugs?

Notes:

44. How/when do I get test results?

Notes:

45. Does my plan cover the Pembrolizumab prescription drugs I need?

Notes:

46. So, are Pembrolizumab prescription drugs safe?

Notes:

47. When does this Pembrolizumab medication expire?

Notes:

48. Does my condition have to be treated with Pembrolizumab prescription drugs?

Notes:

49. Should I take medication to lower my blood pressure?

Notes:

50. Can people be guilty of DUI if they are driving under the influence of Pembrolizumab prescription medications?

Notes:

51. What herbs, supplements, foods, drinks or activities should I avoid while taking Pembrolizumab medication?

Notes:

52. When I have been on the same amount of Pembrolizumab medication for years – when should that be re-evaluated?

Notes:

53. Can Pembrolizumab prescription drugs cause problems during pregnancy?

Notes:

54. What medications do I need to stop and when?

Notes:

55. What does one do when the only real help, the only Pembrolizumab medication available, no longer works?

Notes:

56. Which of my medications cause the most weight gain?

Notes:

57. What happens if I am willing to try new medications if the current Pembrolizumab ones are not working?

Notes:

58. Where are Pembrolizumab prescription drug users getting their prescription filled locally?

Notes:

59. Is it legal to buy Pembrolizumab prescription medications online?

Notes:

60. How do I deal with any Pembrolizumab prescription medication when a side effect may be stated as 'may cause nausea or vomiting'?

Notes:

61. When will I know that I am taking excessive pain medication?

Notes:

62. Can all doctors prescribe Pembrolizumab Prescription Medication?

Notes:

63. Is the answer in natural supplements, in Pembrolizumab prescription medications or some combination of both?

Notes:

64. Will Pembrolizumab interact with any other medicines I take - including any vitamins - herbal medicine or other complementary medicine?

Notes:

65. Can I expect any side effects from my Pembrolizumab medication?

Notes:

66. Can Reiki be used when taking Pembrolizumab medications?

Notes:

67. Will I be able to take my prescription medications after surgery?

Notes:

68. Are my Pembrolizumab medications safe to use while breastfeeding?

Notes:

69. If you have a Pembrolizumab prescription drug in your pocket, outside of the container when arrested is that considered DUI?

Notes:

70. Is Pembrolizumab medication a substitute for therapy?

Notes:

71. What if I start depending on antidepressants, alcohol, or other medications to calm me down or help me sleep?

Notes:

72. When should I stop taking Pembrolizumab medication?

Notes:

73. Should I eat while taking specialized Pembrolizumab prescription drugs?

Notes:

74. When should I take this Pembrolizumab medicine?

Notes:

75. Are there any supplements or Pembrolizumab medications?

Notes:

76. Will Pembrolizumab have an effect on nausea?

Notes:

77. Can I take the generic version of your prescription drugs?

Notes:

78. What should I do if my symptoms are not relieved while taking Pembrolizumab medication?

Notes:

79. Is Pembrolizumab addictive?

Notes:

80. What if I take pain medication for _____?

Notes:

81. Can I take _____ with Pembrolizumab prescription drugs?

Notes:

82. When did you graduate from medical school?

Notes:

83. Are there any known Pembrolizumab prescription medication and chia seeds side effects when they are combined?

Notes:

84. Could natural products be just as effective as Pembrolizumab prescription medications?

Notes:

85. Will I need any Pembrolizumab medication after

surgery?

Notes:

86. How and when should I take my Pembrolizumab medication?

Notes:

87. Are the supplements I take worthwhile?

Notes:

88. Is Pembrolizumab a slow releasing medication?

Notes:

89. How do prescription medications compare to herbal forms of treatment for my condition?

Notes:

90. Is it either / or when it comes to natural medicines and Pembrolizumab prescription drugs?

Notes:

91. Could Pembrolizumab prescription medications cause a false positive on a test?

Notes:

92. Are there any counter-indications about taking this supplement while taking any prescription drugs?

Notes:

93. Does switching Pembrolizumab prescription drugs to over the counter as I age have any negative side effects?

Notes:

CHAPTER #5: WHY:

INTENT: Why do I need Pembrolizumab
(Are there Alternatives. Why do I need
it. Which symptoms does it medicate.)

1. Can using too much or too little Pembrolizumab
prescription drugs harm my health?

Notes:

2. Why can't I buy some prescription drugs online?

Notes:

3. Which medication for my condition is right for me?

Notes:

4. Can a Pembrolizumab prescription drug card preserve me cash?

Notes:

5. Will Pembrolizumab interact with my current medications?

Notes:

6. How do you handle potential prescription drug addiction and flow-on depression?

Notes:

7. Why would I, while regularly taking prescription medications, have to approach grapefruit consumption with caution?

Notes:

8. Are nutritional supplements safe to take if I am taking Pembrolizumab prescription medications?

Notes:

9. Do vitamins interact with Pembrolizumab medications?

Notes:

10. Are herbal supplements safe when I am taking other Pembrolizumab prescription medications?

Notes:

11. When is it time to think about why I'm on these Pembrolizumab drugs?

Notes:

12. Are there any contraindications with Pembrolizumab to other medications?

Notes:

13. Why are we doing these tests?

Notes:

14. Why do I need Pembrolizumab medicine?

Notes:

15. Why does a prescription drug require authorization by a qualified professional and others do not?

Notes:

16. Can the Pembrolizumab medication cause substance abuse?

Notes:

17. Why and when use acupuncture for treating pain instead of, or combined with, taking pain medication?

Notes:

18. Can you help me save money on my Pembrolizumab prescription medication?

Notes:

19. Should I have a current emergency contact

form and a list of health conditions and medications readily available?

Notes:

20. If I take a Pembrolizumab medication, will it require more medication to counter the side effects?

Notes:

21. Which Pembrolizumab medications are addictive?

Notes:

22. Will Pembrolizumab prescription medications cause weight loss?

Notes:

23. Is this worth getting Pembrolizumab medication for?

Notes:

24. Are all Pembrolizumab prescription drugs covered under health care plans?

Notes:

25. Is there a better way to easily adhere to Pembrolizumab prescription medication regimens?

Notes:

26. If I take Pembrolizumab prescription drugs long term, do I run the risk of becoming addicted?

Notes:

27. Will Pembrolizumab meet my expectations?

Notes:

28. Why are you doing this test?

Notes:

29. Will Pembrolizumab interfere with other prescription medications?

Notes:

30. Are there any drug interactions if Pembrolizumab is taken in combination with other medications?

Notes:

31. If I am taking Pembrolizumab prescription medications can I take natural remedies?

Notes:

32. Will I get possible side neuritis of Pembrolizumab medications?

Notes:

33. Why are Pembrolizumab medications so popular?

Notes:

34. Do I have to be on more medications because of the side effects of Pembrolizumab?

Notes:

35. Does the Pembrolizumab medicine need to be stored in the fridge?

Notes:

36. Can nutritional yeasts, especially brewers yeast, interact with Pembrolizumab medications?

Notes:

37. Is there an effective herbal alternative or supplement to Pembrolizumab medication?

Notes:

38. Will I be able to do _____ after treatment?

Notes:

39. Why is Pembrolizumab a prescription drug?

Notes:

40. Do individual policies pay for prescription Pembrolizumab medications?

Notes:

41. Are there any co-pays for medical treatments, hospitalization or Pembrolizumab prescription drugs?

Notes:

42. May an employer ask all employees what prescription medications they are taking?

Notes:

43. Why do I need to manage Pembrolizumab medications?

Notes:

44. What if I am currently without prescription drug coverage?

Notes:

45. Have you instructed patients to discontinue taking their Pembrolizumab, or other prescription drugs?

Notes:

46. Do I need any Pembrolizumab medications?

Notes:

47. What if I refuse the prescribed Pembrolizumab medication?

Notes:

48. What is a 3-Tier or 4-Tier prescription drug plan?

Notes:

49. Are Pembrolizumab prescription drugs covered?

Notes:

50. Why is this Pembrolizumab medication prescribed?

Notes:

51. Why are you giving me a blood test - and what will the results tell us?

Notes:

52. Why is Pembrolizumab medication prescribed?

Notes:

53. Will any supplements interact with my Pembrolizumab prescription drugs?

Notes:

54. How does herb _____ compare to, or has an effect on, Pembrolizumab prescription drugs?

Notes:

55. Can I ever be free of having to use prescription drugs?

Notes:

56. What should I consider when buying coverage that provides prescription drug benefits?

Notes:

57. Are any medications I am taking dangerous for my stage of this disease?

Notes:

58. Should I get a second opinion?

Notes:

59. Are there any other restrictions on Pembrolizumab prescription drug coverage?

Notes:

60. What is the safest prescription drug disposal method?

Notes:

61. How does a Pembrolizumab medication reminder service work?

Notes:

62. Is there an Over-The-Counter Medication that helps or maybe even can replace my Pembrolizumab Prescription Medication?

Notes:

63. Should I stop taking my Pembrolizumab medication(s) before a evaluation or a surgery?

Notes:

64. Why is buying Pembrolizumab prescription drugs without a prescription dangerous?

Notes:

65. Will I have to take my medications forever?

Notes:

66. Is there anything I should do to help prevent my health issue?

Notes:

67. Why have my bowel habits/appetite/mood/sex drive/etc changed?

Notes:

68. If I am stranded abroad and run out of my normal Pembrolizumab prescription medication, am I covered for this?

Notes:

69. Is it necessary to refill my Pembrolizumab medication repeatedly annually?

Notes:

70. Is Pembrolizumab as effective as other prescription medications?

Notes:

71. Why go the Pembrolizumab medication route?

Notes:

72. Will my gender or ethnic group be denied Pembrolizumab medications that work better for other groups but not for my ethnic or gender group?

Notes:

73. Should I buy generic Pembrolizumab prescription medications?

Notes:

74. Are all Pembrolizumab drugs covered by my prescription drug benefit?

Notes:

75. Is it okay to take my Pembrolizumab prescription drugs and multivitamin during a fast?

Notes:

76. Where can US citizens buy their prescription drugs online from legally, in confidence, and under which conditions?

Notes:

77. What medications are safe for me to take during my pregnancy?

Notes:

78. Are extended-release (ER) opioid medications optimum pain medications?

Notes:

79. Is it probable to uncover how to deal with _____ without taking prescription medication?

Notes:

80. Could you write it down?

Notes:

81. Should I expect a dependance on a medication which provides relief?

Notes:

82. I am on prescription Pembrolizumab medication, can I still detox?

Notes:

83. How will the treatment effect the medications that I currently take for _____?

Notes:

84. Has anyone ever used this Pembrolizumab medication?

Notes:

85. Do I really need this treatment?

Notes:

86. Why does my family's medical history matter, and what should I do about it?

Notes:

87. Should I take Pembrolizumab medication or explore alternative natural treatments?

Notes:

88. Will my Pembrolizumab prescription drugs build up toxins in my body?

Notes:

89. Why would I need Pembrolizumab prescription medication reminders?

Notes:

90. How long will I need to take this Pembrolizumab medication?

Notes:

91. Why is it important to take my Pembrolizumab prescription medication exactly as prescribed?

Notes:

92. Are there safe Pembrolizumab-class prescription drugs available?

Notes:

93. Should I bring my Pembrolizumab medications with me everywhere I go?

Notes:

CHAPTER #6: HOW:

INTENT: How will Pembrolizumab affect
me (How will it affect me negatively.
How do I know if its a problem for me.)

1. How can I reduce or stop some of my medications?

Notes:

2. How do I dispose of Pembrolizumab prescription medications?

Notes:

3. Should I bring a copy of my prescription medications?

Notes:

4. How can Pembrolizumab prescription drug abuse be recognized and stopped?

Notes:

5. How long will it take to get the results?

Notes:

6. Can I take Pembrolizumab medication?

Notes:

7. How effective is this treatment?

Notes:

8. Which prescription medications can cause impotence?

Notes:

9. How soon do I need to have the test?

Notes:

10. How wide-ranging is the Pembrolizumab prescription drug coverage?

Notes:

11. How should I take this Pembrolizumab medication?

Notes:

12. How long does the Pembrolizumab medication last?

Notes:

13. How will Pembrolizumab affect the other medications that I'm taking?

Notes:

14. So how do you know if you, or someone you love is having problems with Pembrolizumab prescription drug abuse?

Notes:

15. Are there support groups for people with this problem and how would I contact them?

Notes:

16. How do generic medications compare in quality to brand name drugs?

Notes:

17. How is the test done?

Notes:

18. How quickly do I have to start the treatment?

Notes:

19. How serious is this condition?

Notes:

20. How do I take this Pembrolizumab medication?

Notes:

21. How long do I need to take the Pembrolizumab medicine for?

Notes:

22. How do different Pembrolizumab-class prescription medications work differently?

Notes:

23. How long do I have to take Pembrolizumab medication?

Notes:

24. What if I am affected by anxiety and don't like the thought of taking prescription medications?

Notes:

25. How long is it likely to last?

Notes:

26. How is the Pembrolizumab medication delivered?

Notes:

27. Do you know how long it will take me to get my Pembrolizumab medication?

Notes:

28. How common is Pembrolizumab prescription drug abuse?

Notes:

29. How should I use this Pembrolizumab medication?

Notes:

30. How long does the prescription drug Pembrolizumab stay in your system?

Notes:

31. How's my weight?

Notes:

32. How will Pembrolizumab affect my sleeping pattern?

Notes:

33. How long should I take Pembrolizumab medication?

Notes:

34. Is Pembrolizumab compatible with my current prescribed medication?

Notes:

35. How often do I need to have the test done?

Notes:

36. How often will I take the Pembrolizumab medication?

Notes:

37. How are Pembrolizumab prescription drugs abused?

Notes:

38. How to store Pembrolizumab medication?

Notes:

39. How long will I need the treatment for?

Notes:

40. How can Pembrolizumab medication be detected?

Notes:

41. How will I feel when I'm on Pembrolizumab medications?

Notes:

42. Where I can get a Pembrolizumab prescription drug?

Notes:

43. How can I support my bone health naturally with and without medication?

Notes:

44. How will I know if the Pembrolizumab prescription and over-the-counter medications I take are interacting properly?

Notes:

45. How many surgeries do you perform each year?

Notes:

46. How can I learn more about my symptoms or condition?

Notes:

47. Do you know of any natural medication to help?

Notes:

48. Is it probable to find out how to deal with my condition without taking Pembrolizumab prescription drugs?

Notes:

49. How will I know if my current Pembrolizumab Prescription Drug coverage is as good as the new Medicare Pembrolizumab Prescription Drug coverage?

Notes:

50. How soon should I come back?

Notes:

51. How often is the Pembrolizumab medication taken?

Notes:

52. Does it matter at what time I use my Pembrolizumab medication?

Notes:

53. In case I need pain relief, how can I get access to medical cannabis?

Notes:

54. How do the police suspect impairment by Pembrolizumab prescription medication?

Notes:

55. Are there drugs to lift my mood, and how can this be achieved without prescription medications?

Notes:

56. So I got a condition and a Pembrolizumab medication – how am I, as a patient, supposed to manage treatment?

Notes:

57. How is Pembrolizumab medication supposed to help me?

Notes:

58. How should I dispose of Pembrolizumab prescription drugs?

Notes:

59. How do I manage my Pembrolizumab medications?

Notes:

60. How many patients with my condition have you treated?

Notes:

61. How can I dispose of my Pembrolizumab prescription drugs safely?

Notes:

62. How long does a Pembrolizumab medication remain active in your body?

Notes:

63. Will Pembrolizumab cause a mood change?

Notes:

64. How do I get better without Pembrolizumab medication?

Notes:

65. How does Pembrolizumab prescription drug abuse start?

Notes:

66. How do I manage multiple prescription medications together with Pembrolizumab?

Notes:

67. Should I take Pembrolizumab with other medications?

Notes:

68. How can I find a few methods that can help my condition without the use of Pembrolizumab prescription medication?

Notes:

69. How does Pembrolizumab interact with other medications?

Notes:

70. How do I know if I have permanent hair loss due to medication?

Notes:

71. How does a person with dementia, living alone, manage her Pembrolizumab medication?

Notes:

72. How can I opt for the generic alternative Pembrolizumab medication that gives me the exact same results?

Notes:

73. Is my weight okay?

Notes:

74. State prescription drug price web sites, how useful are they to me as a Pembrolizumab consumer?

Notes:

75. How can I reduce my Pembrolizumab prescription drug costs?

Notes:

76. How do I read the label on my Pembrolizumab prescription drug package?

Notes:

77. How about a new Pembrolizumab-like

prescription drug?

Notes:

78. How should this Pembrolizumab medication be stored?

Notes:

79. How will I get the test results?

Notes:

80. So how do I save money on my Pembrolizumab prescription drugs?

Notes:

81. How to go about it if I want to use a lower dosage of Pembrolizumab?

Notes:

82. How long will the effect of Pembrolizumab medication last?

Notes:

83. How can my mental state successfully improve using medication or therapy?

Notes:

84. How do we order or pick up Pembrolizumab medications?

Notes:

85. My Pembrolizumab medications, just how safe are they?

Notes:

86. How accurate are the results of the test?

Notes:

87. How will I hear about my test results?

Notes:

88. How can I make sure I am sufficiently stocked with the Pembrolizumab prescription medications I need?

Notes:

89. Is this necessary right now?

Notes:

90. Is there a certain Pembrolizumab or other medication that can improve my symptoms?

Notes:

91. How do you handle children on Pembrolizumab medication?

Notes:

92. How should I take my Pembrolizumab medication?

Notes:

93. How should this Pembrolizumab medication be taken?

Notes:

CHAPTER #7: HOW MUCH:

INTENT: How much will taking Pembrolizumab cost me (In money and Pembrolizumab's effect on quality of life.)

1. Is it covered by Medicare - my concession or Veterans Affairs card or my private health insurance?

Notes:

2. Am I am worrying too much?

Notes:

3. Does my policy cover Pembrolizumab prescription drugs?

Notes:

4. Can I take Pembrolizumab with my current medications?

Notes:

5. So, is this a 'wow-factor' Pembrolizumab medication?

Notes:

6. Is sharing Pembrolizumab prescription drugs illegal?

Notes:

7. Regarding dosage, exactly how much of Pembrolizumab can I take?

Notes:

8. Should I join a Medicare Prescription Drug Plan even if I don't take many prescription drugs?

Notes:

9. Is Pembrolizumab safe if taking medications for high blood pressure?

Notes:

10. Do Pembrolizumab medications accelerate aging?

Notes:

11. How much do I need to really understand about the interactions of my Pembrolizumab prescription drugs?

Notes:

12. Are there other remedies, is there any relief other than Pembrolizumab Medication?

Notes:

13. How can you help me when I suffer from chronic pain, but am leery about taking prescription medication to help it?

Notes:

14. How much will the treatment cost?

Notes:

15. Could I have afforded it without Pembrolizumab prescription drug insurance?

Notes:

16. Are there any risks involved in having this test?

Notes:

17. May I bring multiple prescription medications to take while I am in custody?

Notes:

18. How long am I expected to take this Pembrolizumab medication?

Notes:

19. Will it help when I tell you about all my current

medications and vitamin and herbal supplements?

Notes:

20. Can you help me with finding the money to purchase doctor visits and also Pembrolizumab prescriptions medication?

Notes:

21. Do generic medications have the exact same ingredients?

Notes:

22. I'm taking prescription medication abroad, will this be covered if it is lost or I run out?

Notes:

23. How can I legally purchase Pembrolizumab prescription medications from Canada?

Notes:

24. Should I take my Pembrolizumab medications at a

regular time each day?

Notes:

25. Can natural be just as potent, if not more potent than over-the-counter drugs, creams and ointments?

Notes:

26. Can certain over the counter medications or Pembrolizumab prescription medications cause a false positive for illegal drugs in a blood test?

Notes:

27. How much can I use this Pembrolizumab prescription drug plan?

Notes:

28. How much does it normally cost to get the surgery done, including all Pembrolizumab medications and tests (ultrasounds,x-rays,medicines, hospital stay)?

Notes:

29. How much will it cost, will the cost be covered by the PBS - my concession or Veterans Affairs card or by private health insurance?

Notes:

30. How much does Pembrolizumab cost?

Notes:

31. Should I be on Pembrolizumab medication?

Notes:

32. How do I know how much my Pembrolizumab prescription medication will be?

Notes:

33. Is there financial help for Pembrolizumab prescription drugs?

Notes:

34. Will Medicare be enough to cover the cost of my

medical care, especially Pembrolizumab prescription drugs?

Notes:

35. Is the Pembrolizumab medication safe?

Notes:

36. How does my child at an out-of-state school obtain prescription drugs?

Notes:

37. Common side effects of Pembrolizumab include?

Notes:

38. Is it safe getting pregnant while on Pembrolizumab medications?

Notes:

39. Are my prescription drugs also available in a generic version?

Notes:

40. How much should I be charged for my Pembrolizumab prescription medications?

Notes:

41. How do I get the Medicare Pembrolizumab prescription drug benefit?

Notes:

42. Do I need to see any other health professionals - such as specialists - physiotherapists - dieticians or dentists?

Notes:

43. Just how much do you know about the numerous types of Pembrolizumab medications for the different types of my condition?

Notes:

44. Would using Pembrolizumab mean that I would need my other medications less?

Notes:

45. What are the Pembrolizumab prescription drug prices?

Notes:

46. What do each of these Pembrolizumab prescription medications have in common?

Notes:

47. How much do the Pembrolizumab prescription drugs cost in this plan as compared to other plans?

Notes:

48. Precisely what are some good reasons Pembrolizumab prescription drugs can be recommended?

Notes:

49. Do I need to take Pembrolizumab medications?

Notes:

50. Are Pembrolizumab medications toxic?

Notes:

51. How to get my Pembrolizumab medication increased?

Notes:

52. Can I take ayurvedic products with Pembrolizumab prescription medications?

Notes:

53. Do some Pembrolizumab prescription drugs cost more or have additional requirements for coverage?

Notes:

54. Do I HAVE to be on Pembrolizumab medication?

Notes:

55. What if my current Pembrolizumab prescription drugs are not on the formulary or are limited on the formulary?

Notes:

56. Are the brands of Pembrolizumab prescription drugs I take covered?

Notes:

57. What is the difference between a natural herbal supplement and a prescription drug?

Notes:

58. Are there other ways to treat my condition?

Notes:

59. Can I use this app I found?

Notes:

60. What does 50 deductible for brand name

prescription drugs mean?

Notes:

61. Is it likely to get worse, or is it likely to get better?

Notes:

62. What should you do if I've messed up with my Pembrolizumab medication?

Notes:

63. Could any of the Pembrolizumab medications contribute to impotence?

Notes:

64. How much Pembrolizumab prescription medication can I order from my pharmacy at one time?

Notes:

65. Which one of Pembrolizumab medications is

better for me than the others?

Notes:

66. Can you explain my options for Medicare, Medicare/Medicaid, Disability, Supplemental Insurance, Part D Prescription Drug Plans, or Medicare Billings?

Notes:

67. Is there a Pembrolizumab prescription drug guide on the internet?

Notes:

68. Will kinesiology interfere with Pembrolizumab medication?

Notes:

69. Pembrolizumab is most definitely a prescription drug?

Notes:

70. May my employer ask me which Pembrolizumab prescription medications I am taking?

Notes:

71. How much will my Pembrolizumab prescription drugs cost me?

Notes:

72. Can I take Pembrolizumab with prescription medication or with an underlying medical condition?

Notes:

73. How much will the plan cover for Pembrolizumab prescription drugs?

Notes:

74. Should I stop taking that Pembrolizumab medication?

Notes:

75. Does my plan have a Pembrolizumab prescription

drug formulary?

Notes:

76. How much will the test cost?

Notes:

77. Who typically, signed up for the Medicare Prescription Drug plan, are already hitting the gap in coverage known as the doughnut hole - and what is my risk of hitting the doughnut hole?

Notes:

78. Is this something I should worry about or is it just a side effect of Pembrolizumab?

Notes:

79. How much am I likely to spend on Pembrolizumab prescription drugs?

Notes:

80. How much experience with this test or

procedure do you have?

Notes:

81. How much will this cost me?

Notes:

82. Will the cost be covered by Medicare - my concession or Veterans Affairs card or by private health insurance?

Notes:

83. Which part of Medicare will cover my Pembrolizumab prescription drugs?

Notes:

84. Is there a Medicare Advantage plan provider who will cover my Pembrolizumab prescription drug costs during the donut hole?

Notes:

85. Are there simpler - safer options?

Notes:

86. How much Pembrolizumab medication can be brought through customs in case I travel?

Notes:

87. Will these Pembrolizumab medications cause weight gain?

Notes:

88. Are there any risks or side effects?

Notes:

89. Is _____ normal to get after only been taking the Pembrolizumab medication for a few days?

Notes:

90. Will any of the supplements that have been prescribed for me interfere with any Pembrolizumab prescription medications I may already be on?

Notes:

91. Can my Pembrolizumab medication be delivered if I don't attend appointments?

Notes:

92. Can the nurse see me?

Notes:

93. How much is Medicare Pembrolizumab prescription drug coverage worth?

Notes:

Index

really   10, 17, 23, 50, 111, 135
reason 5, 21
reasons   43, 50, 142
receive   10, 19-20
receiving   27
recently   3
recognized   115
recommend   32, 38, 45, 53, 62, 68
recording   1
Records   9, 17
recurring   52
reduce80, 114, 128
references   152
refill   108
refuse   104
regarding   1, 7, 134
regimen   9
regimens   100
regular 45-46, 138
regularly   96
reimburse   20
related19, 51
relation   31, 39
releasing   93
relevant   3
relief   27, 55, 68, 110, 124, 135
relieve 66
relieved   91
religion61
remain 126
remedies   28, 46, 59-60, 101, 135
remedy   39
remember   35
remind 79
reminder   106
reminders   20, 82, 112
repeatedly   108
replace   1, 107
reproduced   1
requested   1
requests   62
require 1, 22, 61, 98-99
required   42

Made in the USA
Monee, IL
17 June 2022

98189359R00095